GERD AND ACID REFLUX COOKBOOK

Easy-to-Make Delicious Meals for Heartburn Relief and LPR.

Christiana White

GAIN ACCESS TO MORE BOOKS

TABLE OF CONTENTS.

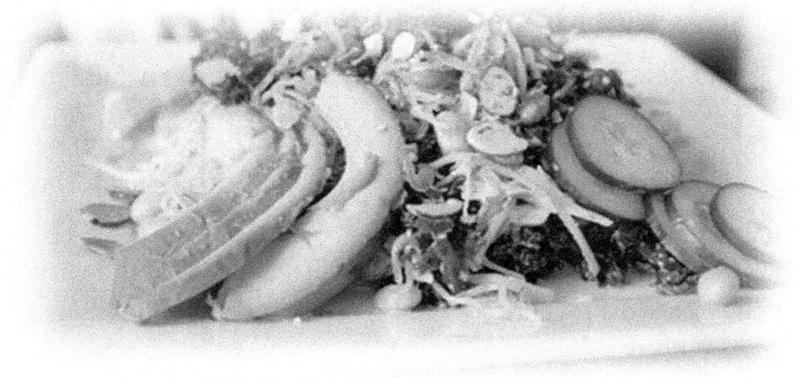

INTRODUCTION

Are you tired of the searing discomfort that acid reflux causes? Do you desire for foods that nourish your body without causing heartburn? Look no further—the Gerd and Acid Reflux Cookbook combines flavor and healing.

We've created a lifeline in these pages, not merely a collection of recipes. Imagine waking up to a calming ginger-infused porridge, eating a light and fulfilling quinoa tabbouleh salad for lunch, then indulging in a lemon herb roasted chicken that won't make you regret a single mouthful. It's not just about what you eat; it's about rediscovering your joy around the dinner table.

But this book is more than simply a compilation of recipes; it's a road map for regaining control of your health and well-being. With insights into trigger foods to avoid, meal planning ideas, and confidence-boosting eating out strategies, you'll see how simple it can be to live a life free of acid reflux.

Dear reader, relief is within grasp. Turn the pages, enjoy the Flavors, and reclaim your life, one meal at a time. Let the Gerd and Acid Reflux Cookbook be your companion on this transformative journey.

Welcome to a world where joy takes precedence over heartburn.

CHAPTER 1

Understand Acid Reflux

Acid reflux, also known as gastroesophageal reflux (GER), is a common digestive problem in which stomach acid backs up into the esophagus, the tube that connects your mouth to your stomach. This acid irritates the esophageal lining, resulting in searing chest pain known as heartburn.

To further comprehend acid reflux, consider the digestive process. When you eat, food passes down the throat by a series of muscle contractions known as peristalsis. The lower esophageal sphincter (LES) is a muscle valve that acts as a one-way gate located at the bottom of the esophagus. Ideally, the LES remains closed except for brief intervals when food and liquids enter into the stomach.

Here's a closer look at the main players:

- **Stomach Acid:** The stomach produces powerful fluids that help break down meals for absorption.
- **Esophagus**: A muscular tube that transports food from the mouth to the stomach.
- **Lower Esophageal Sphincter (LES)**: A muscular valve at the bottom of the esophagus that functions as a one-way gate, stopping stomach contents from flowing back up.

Causes and Triggers for Acid Reflux

Several causes might contribute to a dysfunctional LES and resulting acid reflux:

LES Dysfunction:

- Weakened LES: As time passes, the LES muscle may weaken, making it difficult to remain fully closed.
- Relaxation Issues: The LES may relax abnormally, causing stomach acid to rise even when no food or drink is going through.

Hiatal hernia: This happens when the upper section of the stomach pushes through the diaphragm, the muscle that separates the chest and the abdomen. This increases pressure on the LES, preventing it from properly closing.

Dietary Triggers: Some meals and beverages can weaken the LES or irritate the esophagus, causing acid reflux. Common culprits include:

- Spicy meals contain capsaicin, which irritates the esophagus lining.
- Fatty or fried foods: Slow digestion and may put pressure on the LES.

- Citrus fruits and tomato-based products: Although not naturally acidic in the stomach, their acidity can irritate the esophagus.
- Chocolate and peppermint: Relax the LES, causing stomach acid to increase.
- Alcohol and fizzy drinks might irritate the esophagus and raise stomach acid levels.

Medications: Certain medications, such as:

- Aspirin and ibuprofen (NSAIDs) can irritate the stomach lining and raise acid levels.
- Antidepressants: Some may relax the LES.
- Muscle relaxants might weaken the LES.

Lifestyle factors:

- Pregnancy: Hormonal changes might relax the LES, resulting in acid reflux.
- Being overweight or obese: Excess weight exerts strain on the abdomen, pushing it up and weakening the LES.
- Smoking weakens the LES and irritates the esophagus.

Symptoms & Complications

The most frequent symptom of acid reflux is heartburn, which is a burning chest sensation that can spread to the neck and throat.

However, acid reflux can present in a number of ways, including:

- Regurgitation is a sour or bitter feeling in the mouth caused by stomach acid backing up into the esophagus.
- Acid erosion of teeth: Because the stomach contents are acidic, chronic acid reflux can harm tooth enamel.
- Difficulty swallowing (dysphagia): Can arise when the esophagus becomes irritated or constricted due to prolonged acid reflux.
- Chest pain: While not necessarily associated with heart problems, acid reflux can induce chest pain that resembles angina (chest pain caused by decreased blood flow to the heart).
- Chronic cough: Acid reflux can irritate the airways and cause a chronic cough.
- Worsening asthma symptoms: Acid reflux can irritate the airways, causing wheezing and shortness of breath.
- Sleep disruption: Acid reflux can induce nighttime heartburn and discomfort, resulting in poor sleep quality.

CHAPTER 2

Explaining Gastroesophageal Reflux Disease (GERD)

Gastroesophageal Reflux Disease (GERD) is a chronic digestive condition characterized by frequent and persistent acid reflux. GERD, unlike occasional heartburn, happens more frequently and can have a substantial influence on a person's quality of life.

Here's the breakdown of GERD:

- **Chronic:** The frequency of GERD distinguishes it from occasional acid reflux. GERD is a long-term condition, not a temporary discomfort.
- **Esophageal Lining Damage**: Chronic stomach acid exposure irritates and inflames the esophagus, which can lead to difficulties.
- **Symptoms Other Than Heartburn**: Although heartburn is a common symptom, GERD can also cause chest pain, difficulty swallowing, chronic coughing, and sleep disturbances.

Understanding Heartburn.

Heartburn, the burning chest pain caused by acid reflux, is a defining symptom of GERD. It occurs when stomach acid backs up into the esophagus, irritating the sensitive lining. The burning feeling often begins under the breastbone and spreads upwards to the neck and throat.

- Cause: Stomach acid irritates the esophageal lining.
- Location: Burning feeling behind the breastbone, which can radiate upward in some cases.
- Triggers: Some meals, beverages, medications, and lifestyle choices might cause heartburn.
- Severity: Heartburn symptoms can range from slight pain to severe burning that interferes with regular activities.

Heartburn is a frequent symptom of GERD, but it does not affect everyone with the condition. However, occasional heartburn does not always imply GERD.

Differentiating Acid Reflux from Other Digestive Disorders.

Acid reflux and GERD can occasionally resemble symptoms of other digestive problems. Here is how to differentiate:

• **Peptic Ulcers**: Much like heartburn, peptic ulcers can produce burning sensation in the upper belly. Ulcer discomfort, on the other hand, is more localized and usually occurs on an empty stomach or between meals, whereas heartburn intensifies after eating or lying down.

• **Gallstones**: Gallstones can cause acute upper right abdomen pain that spreads to the back or shoulder blade. This pain varies from the burning sensation associated with acid reflux.

• **Esophageal Cancer**: Although uncommon, esophageal cancer can cause difficulties swallowing, weight loss, and chronic heartburn that does not respond to treatment. This demands quick medical evaluation.

If you have persistent heartburn, difficulty swallowing, or any other troubling symptoms, you should see a doctor to get a proper diagnosis and discuss appropriate treatment choices.

CHAPTER 3

Acid Reflux Diet Basics

Dietary choices can help you manage acid reflux. This chapter delves into the concept of an acid reflux diet, including foods to avoid (triggers and culprits) and meals that are soft on the digestive system.

Foods to Avoid: Trigger Foods and Culprits

Certain foods and beverages may weaken or irritate the lower esophageal sphincter (LES), exacerbating acid reflux symptoms.

• **Fatty and Fried Foods**: High-fat meals impede digestion and exert strain on the LES, causing stomach acid to accumulate more easily. Fried foods, fatty meat cuts, and processed foods high in saturated and harmful fats are some examples.

• **Spicy Foods**: Spices, especially chili peppers with capsaicin, can irritate the esophageal lining and cause heartburn.

• **Citrus Fruits and Tomato-Based Products**: While the stomach is not naturally acidic, the acidity of citrus fruits (oranges, grapefruits, lemons) and tomato-based products (tomato sauce, ketchup) might irritate the esophagus in some people.

• **Chocolate and Peppermint**: Both chocolate and peppermint can relax the LES, making stomach acid rise more easily.

• **Alcohol and carbonated beverages:** Alcohol can irritate the esophagus and raise stomach acid levels. Carbonated drinks can dilate the stomach and put pressure on the LES, exacerbating reflux.

• **Caffeine**: While the effects vary, caffeine may relax the LES and irritate the stomach in some persons, resulting in heartburn.

• **Mint**: Like peppermint, mint can relax the LES and exacerbate acid reflux.

Additional considerations:

• **Food Intolerances**: Pay close attention to individual food sensitivities. Even while onions, garlic, and dairy products are generally well-tolerated, some persons may have heartburn.

• **Portion Control**: Overeating can extend the stomach and put pressure on the LES, causing reflux. Eat smaller, more frequent meals throughout the day.

Foods To Enjoy That Are Gentle on The Digestive System

Variety of food options can help manage acid reflux by boosting healthy digestion and reducing irritation:

• **Lean Protein Sources**: Grilled chicken, fish, and beans are low in fat and easy to digest, reducing the pressure on the digestive system.

• **Whole Grains**: Whole grains such as brown rice, quinoa, and whole-wheat bread contain complex carbs that digest slowly, increasing satiety and relieving strain on the LES.

• **Fruits and vegetables (with a few exceptions)**: Most fruits and vegetables are ideal for an acid reflux diet. Choose non-citrus fruits, such as melons, bananas, and apples. Green beans, broccoli, and carrots are terrific choices.

• **Healthy Fats**: Olive oil, avocado, almonds, and seeds can all provide health benefits. They increase satiety and may lower stomach acid production. However, moderation is essential, since excessive fat intake might aggravate reflux.

• **Ginger**: Ginger contains anti-inflammatory qualities that may soothe the esophagus and relieve heartburn symptoms. However, it might have varying effects on various people, so be careful how you respond.

• **Water**: Staying hydrated is critical. Water dilutes stomach acid and supports proper digestion.

Remember:

- Individual triggers can differ. It is critical to understand your specific food sensitivities and modify your diet accordingly.
- Keeping a food journal to record meals and subsequent heartburn symptoms can help identify causes.

By following an acid reflux diet that focuses on mild, easily digestible meals and avoiding known triggers, you can greatly enhance your digestive comfort and effectively control your acid reflux symptoms.

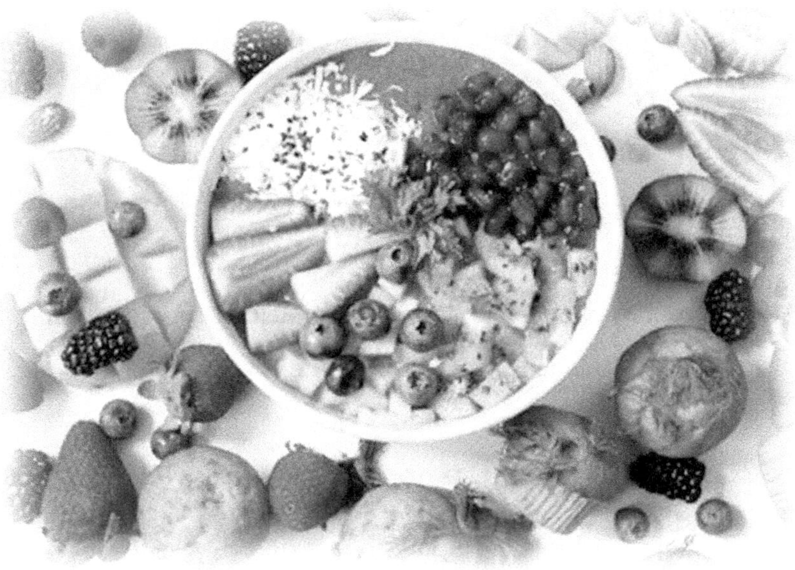

CHAPTER 4

Cooking Methods for Acid Reflux

Living with acid reflux does not imply forsaking good meals. This chapter delves into light cooking methods that are easy on the digestive system, alternative seasonings to reduce discomfort, and helpful tips and tactics for making delicious and reflux-friendly meals.

Light Cooking Techniques for Digestive Ease

Certain cooking methods are gentler on your digestive system than others. Here are some reflux-friendly techniques to consider:

- **Baking and Broiling**: These dry-heat methods use little oil or fat, easing the burden on your digestive system. Baked or grilled chicken, fish, and veggies are wonderful options.

- **Poaching and Steaming:** Both poaching (cooking in a simmering liquid) and steaming utilize little water or broth to gently cook food, retaining nutrients and reducing fat content. Poached fish, poultry, and steamed veggies are all healthful and reflux-friendly choices.

- **Grilling**: Grilling helps excess fat to drain while imparting a Smokey taste. Grilling is ideal for lean cuts of meat, fish, and vegetables. However, be cautious of charring, which can cause irritation.

Techniques to Minimize:

- Frying: Fried foods are heavy in fat and may exacerbate reflux symptoms. Choose healthier cooking methods whenever possible.
- Sautéing: Sautéing is often healthier than frying, but use very little oil.

Seasoning Without Irritation.

Spices and herbs can enhance the flavor of your meals, but some may irritate the esophagus. Here are some reflux-friendly alternatives:

• **Limit**: Spicy peppers, chili powder, cayenne pepper, and black pepper may be triggers. Consider milder options, such as paprika or smoked paprika.

• **Alternatives**: Fresh herbs such as basil, rosemary, thyme, and parsley enhance flavor without causing irritation. Instead of whole citrus fruits, consider using lemon juice or zest to add some acidity.

• **Ginger and Garlic (with Caution):** Ginger and garlic have anti-inflammatory compounds that may aid certain people. However, they can exacerbate symptoms in others. Introduce them gradually and observe your reaction.

• **Salt in moderation**: Too much sodium can aggravate bloating, a frequent reflux symptom. Rather than relying entirely on salt, add flavor using herbs and spices.

• **Acidic substances**: Be cautious of acidic substances such as tomatoes, vinegar, and citrus juices. Use them sparingly, or substitute low-acid alternatives such as cooked tomatoes.

Tips for Acid Reflux-Friendly Cooking

- Thickeners: To provide a soothing consistency, thicken sauces and soups with cornstarch, arrowroot powder, or mashed potatoes.
- Smaller Meals: Eat smaller, more frequent meals throughout the day to avoid overeating and relieve strain on the LES.
- Stay Upright After Eating: Avoid lying down straight after eating. Stay upright for at least 2-3 hours to allow food to properly digest and avoid reflux.

- Mindful Eating: Eat deliberately and relish your meals. Chewing deeply improves digestion and lowers the risk of heartburn.

You may make delicious and satisfying meals without triggering your acid reflux by adopting these culinary techniques, seasoning options, and helpful advice.

Remember that individual sensitivities may vary. Experiment with various ways and components to determine which works best for you.

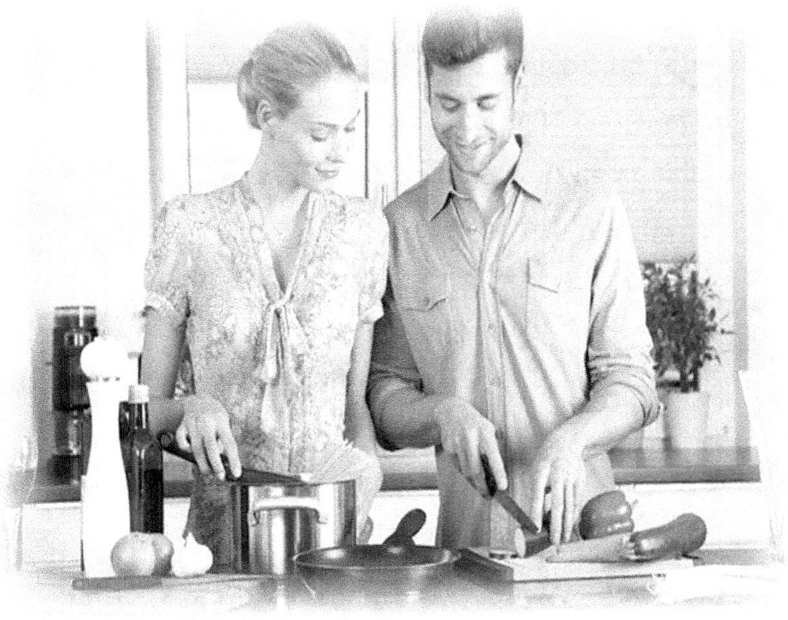

CHAPTER 5

Breakfasts to Begin Your Day Right

Banana Oatmeal Smoothie

- *Servings: Two.*
- *Prep time: 5 minutes.*

Ingredients:

- One ripe banana.
- 1/2 cup rolled oats.
- 1 cup almond milk, unsweetened
- 1/2 teaspoon of ground cinnamon.
- 1 tablespoon honey (optional, based on tolerance).
- 1/2 cup plain Greek yogurt.

Instructions:

- Place the rolled oats in a blender and process until finely powdered.
- Place the ripe banana, almond milk, ground cinnamon, and Greek yogurt in the blender.
- Blend until smooth. If the recipe is too thick, add a little more almond milk until you get the ideal consistency.

- Taste and add honey as desired, as long as it does not cause acid reflux.
- Pour into glasses and serve immediately.

Nutritional Information (Per Serving):

- Calories: 210.
- Protein: 8 grams
- Dietary fibre: 4g

Pear and Spinach Green Smoothie

- *Serves: 1*
- *Prep time: 5 minutes.*

Ingredients:

- One ripe pear, cored and sliced
- 1 cup fresh spinach leaves.
- 1/2 banana (optional for extra sweetness)
- One cup unsweetened almond milk.
- One pinch of ground ginger.

Instructions:

- In a blender, combine the pear, spinach leaves, banana (optional), almond milk, and ground ginger.
- Blend until smooth and creamy.

- Taste and adjust the sweetness, adding honey as needed and tolerated.
- Serve immediately for optimal flavor and nutritional retention.

Nutritional Information (Per Serving):

- Calories: 150.
- Protein: 2 grams
- Dietary fibre: 5g

Ginger-Infused Overnight Oats

- ***Serves: 1***
- ***Preparation time: eight hours (overnight).***

Ingredients:

- 1/2 cup rolled oats.
- 3/4 cup almond milk, unsweetened
- 1/4 teaspoon of ground ginger.
- One spoonful of chia seeds.
- 1/2 apple, grated
- One pinch of cinnamon (optional)

Instructions:

- In a mason jar or dish, mix together the rolled oats, almond milk, ground ginger, and chia seeds.
- Stir in the grated apple and a dash of cinnamon, if preferred.
- Cover and refrigerate overnight.
- In the morning, mix the oats thoroughly. If they're too thick, add a little extra almond milk.
- Serve cold or warm up for a pleasant breakfast.

Nutritional Information (Per Serving):

- *Calories: 250.*
- *Protein: 6 grams*
- *Dietary fibre: 7g*

Avocado Toast with Poached Eggs.

- ***Serves: 1***
- ***Prep time: 10 minutes.***

Ingredients:

- One slice of whole grain bread.
- One-half ripe avocado
- 1 egg
- A dash of paprika (optional).

- Freshly ground black pepper to taste.

Instructions:

- Toast the whole grain bread to your preference.
- Mash the avocados and spread them on bread.
- Poach the egg to your preferred doneness and set it on top of the avocado.
- Season with a pinch of paprika and black pepper to taste.
- Serve immediately and enjoy!

Nutritional Information (Per Serving):

- *Calories: 300.*
- *Protein: 10 grams.*
- *Dietary fibre: 5g*

Quinoa Porridge with Apples and Cinnamon.

- ***Servings: Two.***
- ***Prep time: 15 minutes.***

Ingredients:

- 1/2 cup washed quinoa.
- One cup of water.
- one apple, peeled and diced
- 1/2 teaspoon of ground cinnamon.

- One-quarter cup almond milk

- 1 tablespoon of maple syrup (optional).

Instructions:

- In a saucepan, heat the quinoa and water until boiling.

- Reduce the heat to low, cover, and simmer for 10 minutes.

- Stir in the diced apple and cinnamon, and simmer until the quinoa is soft and the water is absorbed.

- Cook for a further 2 minutes after adding the almond milk and, if using, maple syrup.

- Serve warm and enjoy!

Nutritional Information (Per Serving):

- *Calories: 220.*

- *Protein: 6 grams*

- *Dietary fibre: 5g*

Almond Butter and Banana Pancakes

- ***Servings: Two.***

- ***Prep time: 20 minutes.***

Ingredients:

- One ripe banana, mashed

- 2 eggs

- One-quarter cup almond butter
- One-half teaspoon baking powder
- One pinch of salt.
- Coconut oil for cooking.

Instructions:

- In a mixing basin, combine the mashed banana, eggs, almond butter, baking powder, and salt thoroughly.
- Heat a nonstick pan over medium heat and add a small amount of coconut oil.
- Pour little amounts of batter into the pan to make pancakes.
- Cook until bubbles appear on the surface, then flip and cook the second side until golden brown.
- If desired, drizzle with honey or maple syrup while still hot.

Nutritional Information (Per Serving):

- *Calories: 315.*
- *Protein: 10 grams.*
- *Dietary fibre: 4g*

Baked Pears with Honey and Walnuts.

- _**Servings: Two.**_
- _**Prep time: 30 minutes.**_

Ingredients:

- Two ripe pears, halved and cored
- Two teaspoons of honey (optional).
- 1/4 cup chopped walnuts.
- One pinch of ground cinnamon

Instructions:

- Preheat the oven to 350°F/175°C.
- Arrange the pear halves on a baking sheet, cut side up.
- If using, drizzle with honey and top with chopped walnuts and cinnamon.
- Bake for 20 to 25 minutes, or until the pears are soft.
- Serve warm, perhaps topped with a dollop of Greek yogurt.

Nutritional Information (Per Serving):

- _Calories:180_
- _Protein: 2 grams_
- _Dietary fibre: 5g_

Carrot and Ginger Juice

- *Serves: 1*
- *Prep time: 10 minutes.*

Ingredients:

- Four big, peeled carrots
- 1/2-inch fresh ginger, peeled
- 1/2 cored apple (optional for sweetness).

Instructions:

- Wash the carrots and ginger thoroughly.
- Cut the carrots into manageable bits for the juicer.
- Juice the carrots and ginger together. If you want to include the apple, do so.
- Stir the juice before pouring it into a glass.
- Consume promptly to obtain the maximum nutrients.

Nutritional Information (Per Serving):

- *Calories: 95.*
- *Protein: 2 grams*
- *Dietary fibre: 3 grams*

Multigrain Waffles with Maple Syrup

- ***Servings: Two.***
- ***Prep time: 20 minutes.***

Ingredients:

- One cup multigrain waffle mix.
- 3/4 cup water.
- One tablespoon of coconut oil.
- 1/4 cup of pure maple syrup (optional).

Instructions:

- Preheat your waffle iron per the manufacturer's directions.
- In a bowl, blend the waffle mix, water, and coconut oil until just incorporated.
- Transfer the batter to the waffle iron and cook until golden brown.
- Drizzle with maple syrup if tolerated.

Nutritional Information (Per Serving):

- *Calories: 260*
- *Protein: 6 grams*
- *Dietary fibre: 4g*

Baked Oatmeal Cups with Blueberries

- *Serving size: 6 cups*
- *Prep time: 30 minutes.*

Ingredients:

- Two cups rolled oats.
- One teaspoon of baking powder.
- One-half teaspoon cinnamon
- One cup unsweetened almond milk.
- 1 egg
- 1/4 cup maple syrup (optional).
- One cup blueberry.

Instructions:

- Preheat your oven to 375°F (190°C).
- In a bowl, combine the oats, baking powder, and cinnamon.
- Stir in the almond milk, egg, and maple syrup (if using) until thoroughly blended.
- Gently fold in the blueberries.
- Spoon the batter into muffin cups and bake for 25 minutes, or until firm and golden.
- Let cool before serving.

Nutritional Information (Per Serving):

- *Calories: 150.*

- *Protein: 5 grams.*

- *Dietary fibre: 4g*

Chia Seed Pudding with Almond Milk

- **Servings: Two.**

- **Preparation time: eight hours (overnight).**

Ingredients:

- 1/4 cup of chia seeds.

- One cup unsweetened almond milk.

- 1/2 teaspoon of vanilla extract.

- 1 tablespoon of honey or maple syrup (optional).

Instructions:

- In a bowl, combine the chia seeds, almond milk, and vanilla essence.

- Cover and refrigerate overnight, or at least four hours.

- Stir the pudding, add sweetness if desired, and serve.

Nutritional Information (Per Serving):

- *Calories: 135.*
- *Protein: 4 grams*
- *Dietary fibre: 9g*

Whole Wheat Banana Muffins

- **Servings: 12 muffins.**
- **Prep time: 35 minutes.**

Ingredients:

- Two cups whole wheat flour.
- One teaspoon of baking soda.
- 1/4 teaspoon of salt.
- 1/2 cup unsweetened applesauce.
- 3/4 cup honey or maple syrup (optional).
- 2 eggs
- 3 ripe bananas (mashed)
- One-quarter cup hot water

Instructions:

- Preheat the oven to 325°F (165° C).
- In a large bowl, combine the flour, baking soda, and salt.

- In a separate bowl, add the applesauce, sweetener (if using), eggs, and mashed bananas.
- Add the banana mixture to the flour mixture, stirring just until combined.
- Stir in the hot water until thoroughly combined.
- Scoop the batter into muffin cups and bake for 20-25 minutes, or until a toothpick comes out clean.
- Let cool before serving.

Nutritional Information (Per Serving):

- *Calories:180*
- *Protein: 4 grams*
- *Dietary fibre: 3 grams*

Savory Oatmeal with Avocado

- **Serves: 1**
- **Prep time: 15 minutes.**

Ingredients:

- 1/2 cup rolled oats.
- One cup of water.
- 1/2 ripe avocado sliced
- One pinch of salt.
- Freshly ground black pepper to taste.

Instructions:

- Cook the oats in water according to the package directions.
- Add a pinch of salt and black pepper.
- Top with sliced avocado.
- Serve hot and enjoy this flavourful take on a breakfast favourite.

Nutritional Information (Per Serving):

- *Calories: 250.*
- *Protein: 6 grams*
- *Dietary fibre: 7g*

Apple Cinnamon Breakfast Quinoa

- ***Servings: Two.***
- ***Prep time: 20 minutes.***

Ingredients:

- 1/2 cup washed quinoa.
- One cup of water.
- One apple, diced
- 1/2 teaspoon of ground cinnamon.
- 1/4 cup of unsweetened almond milk.
- 1 tablespoon of honey or maple syrup (optional).

Instructions:

- In a saucepan, combine the quinoa and water and heat till boiling.
- Reduce the heat to low, cover, and simmer for 15 minutes.
- Add the diced apple and cinnamon, and simmer until the apple is tender.
- Remove from the heat and stir in the almond milk and sugar, if desired and tolerated.
- Serve warm and enjoy!

Nutritional Information (Per Serving):

- *Calories: 235.*
- *Protein: 6 grams*
- *Dietary fibre: 6g*

Yogurt Parfait with Mixed Berries.

- ***Serves: 1***
- ***Prep time: 5 minutes.***

Ingredients:

- One cup plain Greek yogurt.
- half cup mixed berries (strawberries, blueberries, raspberries)

- 1 tablespoon of granola (optional).

Instructions:

- In a serving glass, place half of the Greek yogurt.
- Arrange a layer of mixed berries.
- Add another layer of Greek yogurt, then top with the remaining berries.
- Sprinkle granola on top if wanted and tolerated.
- Serve immediately and have a refreshing breakfast.

Nutritional Information (Per Serving):

- *Calories: 190.*
- *Protein: 20 grams*
- *Dietary fibre: 2 grams*

CHAPTER 6

Light And Soothing Lunches.

Grilled Chicken Salad with Balsamic Vinaigrette

- **_Servings: Two._**
- **_Prep time: 20 minutes._**

Ingredients:

- Two boneless and skinless chicken breasts.
- 4 cups mixed greens (lettuce, spinach, and arugula
- 1/2 cup cherry tomatoes, cut in half
- 1/4 cup sliced cucumber.
- 1/4 cup of shredded carrots.
- Two teaspoons of balsamic vinegar.
- One tablespoon of olive oil.
- One teaspoon of honey (optional)
- Add salt and pepper to taste.

Instructions:

- Preheat the grill to medium-high heat.
- Season chicken breasts with salt and pepper, then grill for 6-7 minutes per side.
- Let the chicken rest for a few minutes before slicing it.

- In a large bowl, combine the mixed greens, cherry tomatoes, cucumber, and carrots.
- In a small bowl, combine the balsamic vinegar, olive oil, and honey, if using.
- Drizzle vinaigrette over salad and toss to coat.
- Garnish the salad with grilled chicken slices and serve.

Nutritional Information (Per Serving):

- *Calories: 290.*
- *Protein: 26 grams.*
- *Dietary fibre: 3 grams*

Baked Sweet Potato and Cottage Cheese

- ***Serves: 1***
- ***Prep time: 45 minutes.***

Ingredients:

- One large sweet potato.
- 1/2 cup cottage cheese, low-fat
- A pinch of cinnamon.
- Fresh chives as garnish (optional).

Instructions:

- Preheat your oven to 400°F (200°C).
- Pierce the sweet potato with a fork and set it on a baking pan.
- Bake for 40 to 45 minutes, or until tender.
- Using a fork, split open the sweet potato and fluff the insides.
- Serve with cottage cheese, a sprinkle of cinnamon, and chives if desired.
- Serve warm and enjoy!

Nutritional Information (Per Serving):

- *Calories: 270.*
- *Protein: 15 grams.*
- *Dietary fibre: 4g*

Turkey and Spinach Wrap with Avocado

- *Serves: 1*
- *Prep time: 10 minutes.*

Ingredients:

- One whole wheat wrap.
- Three slices of turkey breast (low sodium)
- 1/2 cup of fresh spinach leaves.
- 1/4 avocado, sliced

* One spoonful plain Greek yogurt.

Instructions:

* Place the wrap flat on a plate.
* Spread the Greek yogurt in the centre of the wrap.
* Place turkey pieces, spinach leaves, and avocado slices on top.
* Roll the wrap securely, then cut in half to serve.

Nutritional Information (Per Serving):

* *Calories: 320.*
* *Protein: 25 grams.*
* *Dietary fibre: 5g*

Butternut Squash Soup

* ***Serves: 4***
* ***Preparation Time: 1 hour.***

Ingredients:

* One medium butternut squash, peeled and cubed
* One tablespoon of olive oil.
* One small onion, chopped
* Four cups of veggie broth.
* Add salt and pepper to taste.

- A pinch of nutmeg, optional.

Instructions:

- Preheat your oven to 375°F (190°C).
- Toss the butternut squash cubes with olive oil and place on a baking pan.
- Roast for 30 minutes or until tender.
- In a pot, cook the onion until transparent.
- Combine the roasted squash and vegetable broth.
- Bring to a simmer, then cook for 20 minutes.
- Puree the soup until smooth, then season with salt, pepper, and nutmeg, if desired.
- Serve hot.

Nutritional Information (Per Serving):

- *Calories:180*
- *Protein: 3 grams.*
- *Dietary fibre: 6g*

<u>*Quinoa Tabbouleh Salad.*</u>

- *Serves: 4*
- *Prep time: 20 minutes.*

Ingredients:

- 1 cup cooked quinoa, cooled
- 1 cup finely chopped parsley.
- 1/2 cup chopped tomatoes.
- 1/2 cup chopped cucumber.
- 2 teaspoons of lemon juice.
- Two teaspoons of olive oil.
- Add salt and pepper to taste.

Instructions:

- In a large mixing bowl, combine the cooked quinoa, parsley, tomatoes, and cucumber.
- In a small bowl, combine the lemon juice, olive oil, salt, and pepper.
- Pour the dressing over the quinoa and toss to incorporate.
- Refrigerate for a minimum of 15 minutes before serving.

Nutritional Information (Per Serving):

- *Calories: 210.*
- *Protein: 6 grams*
- *Dietary fibre: 5g*

Rice Paper Rolls with Mango and Mint.

- *Servings: Two.*
- *Prep time: 30 minutes.*

Ingredients:

- Four rice paper sheets.
- 1/2 thinly sliced mango.
- 1 cup shredded lettuce.
- One-quarter cup mint leaves
- One-quarter cup cooked rice noodles
- 1/4 cup julienned carrots.

Instructions:

- Dip one rice paper sheet into warm water for a few seconds until soft.
- Place the sheet flat on a clean surface and fill with a tiny amount of lettuce, mango, mint, rice noodles, and carrots.
- Fold the rice paper's sides in and roll it up tightly.
- Repeat for the remaining sheets.
- Serve with a side of mild soy sauce or ginger-infused dipping sauce.

Nutritional Information (Per Serving):

- *Calories: 150.*

- *Protein: 2 grams*

- *Dietary fibre: 2 grams*

Baked Falafel with Tahini Sauce

- ***Serves: 4***

- ***Preparation Time: 1 hour.***

Ingredients:

- 2 cups canned chickpeas (drained and rinsed)

- 1/4 cup minced onion.

- 2 garlic cloves, minced

- 2 tablespoons parsley, chopped

- One teaspoon cumin.

- Add salt and pepper to taste.

- Two tablespoons tahini.

- One tablespoon of lemon juice.

- One tablespoon of water.

Instructions:

- Preheat your oven to 375°F (190°C).
- In a food processor, mix together chickpeas, onion, garlic, parsley, cumin, salt, and pepper. Process until evenly blended but not pureed.
- Shape the mixture into tiny patties and transfer to a baking sheet lined with parchment paper.
- Bake for 25–30 minutes, flipping halfway through, until brown and firm.
- To make the sauce, mix together tahini, lemon juice, and water until smooth.
- Drizzle tahini sauce over the falafel before serving.

Nutritional Information (Per Serving):

- *Calories: 260*
- *Protein: 9 grams.*
- *Dietary fibre: 6g*

Lentil Salad with Cucumber and Herbs.

- *Servings: Two.*
- *Prep time: 15 minutes.*

Ingredients:

- One cup cooked lentil.
- 1/2 cucumber, diced
- 1/4 cup fresh parsley, chopped
- 1/4 cup fresh mint, chopped
- 2 teaspoons of lemon juice.
- One tablespoon of olive oil.
- Add salt and pepper to taste.

Instructions:

- In a large bowl, combine the cooked lentils, cucumber, parsley, and mint.
- In a small bowl, combine the lemon juice, olive oil, salt, and pepper.
- Toss the lentil mixture with the dressing until evenly coated.
- Refrigerate for a minimum of 10 minutes before serving.

Nutritional Information (Per Serving):

- *Calories: 240*
- *Protein: 12 grams*
- *Dietary fibre: 9g*

Roasted Beet and Carrot Salad.

- *Servings: Two.*
- *Prep time: 45 minutes.*

Ingredients:

- Two medium beets, peeled and diced
- Two medium carrots, peeled and sliced
- One tablespoon of olive oil.
- Two cups of mixed greens
- Two teaspoons of balsamic vinegar.
- Add salt and pepper to taste.

Instructions:

- Preheat your oven to 400°F (200°C).
- Toss the beets and carrots with olive oil and place on a baking sheet.
- Roast for 30 to 35 minutes, or until soft and lightly caramelized.
- Let the vegetables cool somewhat before tossing with the mixed greens.
- Drizzle with balsamic vinegar, then season with salt and pepper. Serve.

Nutritional Information (Per Serving):

- *Calories:180*

- *Protein: 3 grams.*
- *Dietary fibre: 6g*

<u>*Cauliflower Rice Stir-Fry*</u>

- **Servings: Two.**
- **Prep time: 20 minutes.**

Ingredients:

- Two cups cauliflower rice.
- One tablespoon of olive oil.
- 1/2 cup chopped bell peppers.
- 1/2 cup peas.
- 1/2 cup julienned carrots.
- Two teaspoons low-sodium soy sauce.
- One teaspoon of sesame oil.
- Add salt and pepper to taste.

Instructions:

- Heat the olive oil in a large skillet over medium heat.
- Combine cauliflower rice, bell peppers, peas, and carrots. Stir-fry for 5–7 minutes.
- Drizzle with soy sauce and sesame oil, then season with salt and pepper.
- Stir-fry for another 2-3 minutes, until the vegetables are soft.

- Serve hot.

Nutritional Information (Per Serving):

- *Calories: 160.*
- *Protein: 4 grams*
- *Dietary fibre: 5g*

Broccoli and Cheese Stuffed Potatoes

- **Servings: Two.**
- **Preparation Time: 1 hour.**

Ingredients:

- Two large russet potatoes.
- 1 cup broccoli florets, steamed
- 1/2 cup shredded cheddar cheese (low-fat)
- 1/4 cup Greek yogurt, plain
- Add salt and pepper to taste.

Instructions:

- Preheat your oven to 400°F (200°C).
- Pierce the potatoes with a fork and bake for 50-60 minutes, until cooked.
- Cut each potato in half and scoop out the insides, leaving a thin coating of potato.

- In a bowl, combine the scooped potato, Greek yogurt, salt, and pepper.

- Add the steamed broccoli and half of the cheese.

- Return the mixture to the potato skins and sprinkle with the remaining cheese.

- Bake for another 10 minutes, or until the cheese melts.

- Serve hot.

Nutritional Information (Per Serving):

- *Calories: 290.*

- *Protein: 15 grams.*

- *Dietary fibre: 4g*

Zucchini Noodles with Pesto

- ***Servings: Two.***

- ***Prep time: 15 minutes.***

Ingredients:

- Two medium zucchinis, spiralized

- 1/4 cup basil pesto (see the remark below)

- 1/4 cup cherry tomatoes, halved

- 1 tablespoon of pine nuts (optional).

- Add salt and pepper to taste.

Instructions:

- In a large mixing basin, combine the spiralized zucchini and pesto until well coated.
- Toss in the cherry tomatoes and optional pine nuts.
- Add salt and pepper to taste.
- Serve immediately or refrigerate before serving.

Nutritional Information (Per Serving):

- Calories:180
- Protein: 4 grams
- Dietary fibre: 3 grams

Grilled Fish Tacos with Cabbage Slaw.

- ***Servings: Two.***
- ***Prep time: 30 minutes.***

Ingredients:

- Two white fish fillets (like tilapia or cod)
- Four corn tortillas.
- One cup of shredded cabbage.
- 1/4 cup of diced tomatoes.
- 1/4 cup of thinly sliced red onion.
- One tablespoon of lime juice.

- One tablespoon of olive oil.
- Add salt and pepper to taste.

Instructions:

- Preheat the grill to medium-high.
- Coat the fish fillets with olive oil and season with salt and pepper.
- Grill the fish for 3-4 minutes per side, or until well done.
- In a bowl, combine the cabbage, tomatoes, red onion, and lime juice.
- Heat the tortillas on the grill for about 30 seconds on each side.
- Flake the grilled fish and distribute it among the tortillas.
- Top with cabbage slaw and serve.

Nutritional Information (Per Serving):

- *Calories: 320.*
- *Protein: 25 grams.*
- *Dietary fibre: 5g*

Vegetable Quiche with Oat Crust

- *Serves: 4*
- *Preparation Time: 1 hour.*

Ingredients:

For the crust:

- One cup rolled oats.
- One-quarter cup almond flour
- 1/4 cup of cold water.
- One tablespoon of olive oil.
- One pinch of salt.

For the Filling:

- 1/2 cup broccoli florets, chopped
- 1/2 bell pepper, diced
- 1/4 cup coarsely chopped red onion.
- 4 eggs
- One-half cup almond milk
- Add salt and pepper to taste.
- 1/2 teaspoon of dried thyme.

Instructions:

- Preheat your oven to 375°F (190°C).
- In a food processor, combine the oats, almond flour, water, olive oil, and salt until it forms a dough.
- Press the dough into a pie dish to make the crust.
- Bake the crust for ten minutes.
- In a bowl, combine the eggs, almond milk, salt, pepper, and thyme.
- Sauté the broccoli, bell pepper, and onion until soft, then equally distribute them on the crust.
- Pour the egg mixture over the veggies.
- Bake for 35-40 minutes, or until the quiche has set and the top is lightly brown.
- Allow it to cool for a few minutes before slicing and serving.

Nutritional Information (Per Serving):

- *Calories: 220.*
- *Protein: 11 grams.*
- *Dietary fibre: 4g*

Soba Noodle Salad with Edamame

- ***Servings: Two.***
- ***Prep time: 20 minutes.***

Ingredients:

- Four ounces of soba noodles.
- 1/2 cup edamame, shelled and cooked.
- 1/2 cup julienned cucumber.
- 1/4 cup julienned carrots.
- Two teaspoons low-sodium soy sauce.
- One tablespoon of rice vinegar.
- One teaspoon of sesame oil.
- One teaspoon of honey (optional)
- Sesame seeds as garnish (optional)

Instructions:

- Cook the soba noodles according to the package directions, then rinse with cold water and drain.
- In a large bowl, combine the noodles, edamame, cucumber, and carrots.
- In a small mixing bowl, combine the soy sauce, rice vinegar, sesame oil, and honey, if using.
- Pour the dressing over the noodles and toss to coat.
- Garnish with sesame seeds if desired.

- Serve cold or room temperature.

Nutritional Information (Per Serving):

- *Calories: 320.*
- *Protein: 12 grams*
- *Dietary fibre: 3 grams*

CHAPTER 7

Dinners That Will Not Disappoint.

Baked Salmon with Dill and Lemon

- ***Servings: Two.***
- ***Prep time: 25 minutes.***

Ingredients:

- Two salmon fillets, 6 ounces apiece.
- One tablespoon of olive oil.
- 1 tablespoon fresh dill, chopped
- One lemon, thinly sliced
- Add salt and pepper to taste.

Instructions:

- Preheat your oven to 375°F (190°C).
- Arrange the salmon fillets on a baking pan lined with parchment paper.
- Drizzle olive oil over the fish, then season with salt and pepper.
- Sprinkle the chopped dill over the fillets and garnish with lemon slices.

- Bake for 15-20 minutes, or until salmon flakes easily with a fork.
- Serve hot, and enjoy!

Nutritional Information (Per Serving):

- *Calories: 280.*
- *Protein: 23 grams.*
- *Dietary fibre: 0 grams*

Grilled Turkey Burgers with Oatmeal

- *Serves: 4*
- *Prep time: 30 minutes.*

Ingredients:

- One pound of ground turkey.
- 1/2 cup rolled oats.
- 1 egg
- 1/4 cup coarsely diced onion
- One teaspoon dried thyme.
- Add salt and pepper to taste.
- Whole wheat hamburger buns (optional).

Instructions:

- In a large bowl, combine ground turkey, rolled oats, egg, onion, thyme, salt, and pepper.
- Form the mixture into four patties.
- Preheat the grill to medium-high and lightly oil the grates.
- Grill the patties for 5-7 minutes per side, or until well done.
- If tolerated, serve on whole wheat buns; otherwise, enjoy the patties on their own.

Nutritional Information (per portion, excluding bun):

- Calories: 220.
- Protein: 27 grams.
- Dietary fibre: 1g

Vegetable Stir-Fry with Ginger Sauce.

- *Servings: Two.*
- *Prep time: 20 minutes.*

Ingredients:

- 2 cups of mixed veggies (broccoli, bell peppers, carrots, snap peas).
- One tablespoon of olive oil.
- One teaspoon of grated ginger.

- One chopped garlic clove (optional).
- Two teaspoons low-sodium soy sauce.
- 1 teaspoon cornstarch dissolved in 2 tablespoons of water.

Instructions:

- Heat the olive oil in a large skillet over medium-high heat.
- Stir-fry the mixed vegetables for 5 minutes.
- Cook for another minute, then stir in the grated ginger and minced garlic if using.
- In a small bowl, combine the soy sauce and cornstarch until smooth.
- Pour the sauce over the vegetables and simmer until thickened.
- Serve hot with a serving of brown rice, if tolerated.

Nutritional Information (Per Serving):

- Calories: 150.
- Protein: 4 grams
- Dietary fibre: 3 grams

Lemon-Herb Roasted Chicken

- *Serves: 4*
- ***Preparation Time: 1 hour 30 minutes.***

Ingredients:

- One entire chicken (about 4 pounds).
- One lemon, quartered
- Four sprigs of fresh thyme
- Two teaspoons of olive oil.
- Add salt and pepper to taste.

Instructions:

- Preheat your oven to 375°F (190°C).
- Put the bird in a roasting pan and stuff the cavity with lemon quarters and thyme sprigs.
- Coat the outside of the chicken with olive oil, salt, and pepper.
- Roast for 1 hour and 20 minutes, or until the juices run clear when cut between the leg and thigh.
- Allow the chicken to rest for ten minutes before carving.

Nutritional Information (Per Serving):

- Total calories: 360.
- Protein: 25 grams.
- Dietary fibre: 0 grams

Baked Cod Served with Steamed Broccoli

- _**Servings: Two.**_
- _**Prep time: 30 minutes.**_

Ingredients:

- Two cod fillets, 6 ounces apiece.
- One tablespoon of olive oil.
- One lemon, cut
- Two cups broccoli florets.
- Add salt and pepper to taste.

Instructions:

- Preheat your oven to 400°F (200°C).
- Arrange the fish fillets on a baking pan lined with parchment paper.
- Drizzle olive oil over the cod and season with salt and pepper.
- Garnish each fillet with lemon slices.
- Bake for 15-20 minutes, or until the fish flaked easily with a fork.
- While the cod bakes, cook the broccoli florets until soft.
- Serve baked cod with steamed broccoli on the side.

Nutritional Information (Per Serving):

- *Calories: 200.*

- *Protein: 22 grams*

- *Dietary fibre: 3 grams*

Herb-Crusted Tilapia with Asparagus

- **Servings: Two.**

- **Prep time: 25 minutes.**

Ingredients:

- 2 tilapia fillets, 6 ounces each

- One tablespoon of olive oil.

- 1/2 cup of whole wheat breadcrumbs.

- 1 tablespoon fresh parsley, chopped

- One teaspoon of dried basil

- One teaspoon of dried oregano.

- 2 cups trimmed asparagus.

- Add salt and pepper to taste.

Instructions:

- Preheat your oven to 375°F (190°C).

- In a bowl, combine the breadcrumbs, parsley, basil, and oregano.

- Brush the tilapia fillets with olive oil and then coat with the breadcrumb mixture.
- Arrange the fillets on a baking sheet coated with parchment paper.
- Arrange the asparagus around the fish; drizzle with olive oil, salt, and pepper.
- Bake for 15-20 minutes, or until the tilapia is thoroughly cooked and the asparagus is soft.
- Serve hot.

Nutritional Information (Per Serving):

- *Calories: 230.*
- *Protein: 23 grams.*
- *Dietary fibre: 4g*

Stuffed Bell Peppers with Quinoa

- ***Serves: 4***
- ***Preparation Time: 1 hour.***

Ingredients:

- 4 bell peppers with tops cut off and seeds removed
- 1 cup cooked quinoa.
- 1/2 cup black beans (drained and rinsed)
- 1/2 cup of corn kernels.

- 1/2 cup of diced tomatoes.

- One teaspoon cumin.

- 1/2 teaspoon of garlic powder.

- 1/2 cup shredded cheddar cheese (low fat)

- Add salt and pepper to taste.

Instructions:

- Preheat the oven to 350°F/175°C.

- In a bowl, combine cooked quinoa, black beans, corn, chopped tomatoes, cumin, garlic powder, salt, and pepper.

- Stuff the mixture into the bell peppers and sprinkle with shredded cheese.

- Place the stuffed peppers in a baking sheet and bake for 30-35 minutes, or until they are soft and the cheese has melted.

- Serve hot.

Nutritional Information (Per Serving):

- Calories: 250.

- Protein: 12 grams

- Dietary fibre: 7g

Chicken and Vegetable Skewers

- *Serves: 4*
- *Preparation time: 45 minutes, including marinating time.*

Ingredients:

- Two boneless, skinless chicken breasts cut into cubes
- 1 zucchini, cut into rounds
- 1 bell pepper, sliced into pieces
- 1 red onion, chopped into bits
- Two teaspoons of olive oil.
- One tablespoon of lemon juice.
- One teaspoon of dried oregano.
- Add salt and pepper to taste.

Instructions:

- In a bowl, combine the olive oil, lemon juice, oregano, salt, and pepper.
- Add the chicken cubes to the marinade and refrigerate for at least 30 minutes.
- Preheat the grill to medium-high.
- Thread the chicken and vegetables on skewers, rotating between them.
- Grill the skewers for 10-15 minutes, rotating regularly, until the chicken is thoroughly cooked.

- Serve hot.

Nutritional Information (Per Serving):

- *Calories: 220.*
- *Protein: 26 grams.*
- *Dietary fibre: 2 grams*

Eggplant Parmesan with Low Acid Tomato Sauce

- **Serves: 4**
- **Preparation Time: 1 hour.**

Ingredients:

- 1 large eggplant, cut into half-inch rounds
- 2 cups low-acid tomato sauce, homemade or store-bought.
- 1 cup shredded mozzarella cheese (low fat)
- 1/4 cup grated parmesan cheese.
- One teaspoon of dried basil
- Add salt and pepper to taste.
- Olive oil for brushing.

Instructions:

- Preheat your oven to 375°F (190°C).
- Brush olive oil on both sides of the eggplant slices and season with salt and pepper.

- Transfer the slices to a baking sheet and bake for 20 minutes, flipping halfway through.
- Add a thin layer of tomato sauce to the bottom of a baking dish.
- Spread eggplant slices over the sauce, then top with additional sauce, mozzarella, and Parmesan cheese.
- Repeat the layers until all of the ingredients are utilized, and top with cheese.
- Sprinkle with dried basil and bake for 25-30 minutes, or until the cheese is melted and golden.
- Serve hot.

Nutritional Information (Per Serving):

- *Calories: 200.*
- *Protein: 12 grams*
- *Dietary fibre: 5g*

Roasted Turkey Breast with Sweet Potatoes.

- *Serves: 4*
- *Preparation Time: Two hours.*

Ingredients:

- One turkey breast (about three pounds)
- Two sweet potatoes, peeled and diced

- Two teaspoons of olive oil.

- One teaspoon dried thyme.

- Add salt and pepper to taste.

Instructions:

- Preheat the oven to 325°F (165° C).

- Season the turkey breast with 1 tablespoon olive oil, thyme, salt, and pepper.

- Place the turkey breast in a roasting pan and cook for 1 hour and 30 minutes, or until the internal temperature reaches 165°F (74°C).

- Mix the sweet potato cubes with the remaining olive oil, salt, and pepper.

- Wrap the sweet potatoes around the turkey in the roasting pan for the final 45 minutes of cooking.

- Once cooked, allow the turkey to rest for 10 minutes before slicing.

- Serve the turkey with roasted sweet potatoes on the side.

Nutritional Information (Per Serving):

- Calories: 340.

- Protein: 35 grams.

- Dietary fibre: 3 grams

<u>*Grilled Shrimp with Garlic and Herbs.*</u>

- *Servings: Two.*
- *Prep time: 20 minutes.*

Ingredients:

- 12 large shrimp (peeled and deveined)
- Two teaspoons of olive oil.
- One garlic clove, minced
- 1 tablespoon fresh parsley, chopped
- One teaspoon of dried oregano.
- Add salt and pepper to taste.
- Lemon wedges to serve.

Instructions:

- In a bowl, combine the olive oil, garlic, parsley, oregano, salt, and pepper.
- Add the shrimp and toss to coat.
- Preheat the grill to medium-high.
- Grill the shrimp for 2-3 minutes per side, or until pink and opaque.
- Serve hot, with lemon wedges on the side.

Nutritional Information (Per Serving):

- Calories:180
- Protein: 24 grams

- Dietary fibre: 0 grams

Seared Scallops with Polenta.

- ***Servings: Two.***
- ***Prep time: 30 minutes.***

Ingredients:

- Six large sea scallops.
- 1 cup cornmeal (polenta)
- Two cups of water.
- One tablespoon of olive oil.
- Add salt and pepper to taste.

Instructions:

- In a saucepan, bring water to a boil before gradually whisking in the polenta.
- Reduce the heat to low and stir frequently until the polenta is thick and creamy.
- Season the scallops with salt and pepper.
- Heat olive oil in a pan over high heat, then sear the scallops for 1-2 minutes on each side, or until a golden crust forms.
- Serve the scallops with the polenta.

Nutritional Information (Per Serving):

- Calories: 270.
- Protein: 14 grams
- Dietary fibre: 2 grams

Vegetable Lasagna with Spinach and Ricotta

- **_Serves: 4_**
- **_Preparation Time: 1 hour._**

Ingredients:

- 9 lasagna noodles (cooked)
- 2 cups ricotta cheese (low fat)
- 1 egg
- Two cups of chopped spinach.
- 1 cup shredded mozzarella cheese (low fat)
- Two cups of low-acid tomato sauce
- One teaspoon of dried basil
- Add salt and pepper to taste.

Instructions:

- Preheat your oven to 375°F (190°C).
- In a bowl, combine the ricotta cheese, egg, spinach, salt, and pepper.

- Add a thin layer of tomato sauce to the bottom of a baking dish.
- Spread a layer of noodles over the sauce, then a layer of ricotta mixture, and top with mozzarella.
- Repeat the layers, finishing with the mozzarella on top.
- Sprinkle with dried basil and bake for 30-35 minutes, or until the cheese is melted and golden.
- Allow it to cool for a few minutes before slicing and serving.

Nutritional Information (Per Serving):

- *Calories: 350.*
- *Protein: 22 grams*
- *Dietary fibre: 3 grams*

Pork Tenderloin and Roasted Apples

- ***Serves: 4***
- ***Preparation Time: 1 hour.***

Ingredients:

- One pork tenderloin (around one pound)
- Two apples, cored and sliced
- One tablespoon of olive oil.
- One teaspoon of dried rosemary
- Add salt and pepper to taste.

Instructions:

- Preheat your oven to 375°F (190°C).
- Season the pork tenderloin with salt, pepper, and rosemary.
- Brown the tenderloin on all sides in a pan over medium-high heat, using olive oil.
- Place the tenderloin in a baking dish and surround it with apple slices.
- Roast for 25-30 minutes, until the internal temperature reaches 145°F (63°C).
- Allow the pork to rest for 5 minutes before slicing.
- Serve with roasted apples.

Nutritional Information (Per Serving):

- *Calories: 240*
- *Protein: 24 grams*
- *Dietary fibre: 2 grams*

Wild Rice Pilaf with Mushrooms and Peas.

- _Serves: 4_
- _Prep time: 45 minutes._

Ingredients:

- One cup wild rice.
- Two cups of vegetable broth.
- 1 cup sliced mushrooms.
- 1/2 cup peas.
- One tablespoon of olive oil.
- Add salt and pepper to taste.

Instructions:

- In a saucepan, bring the vegetable broth to a boil, then add the wild rice.
- Reduce the heat to low, cover, and let simmer for 35-40 minutes, or until the rice is tender.
- Heat olive oil in a skillet over medium heat, then sauté the mushrooms until browned.
- Add the peas to the skillet and cook for another 2-3 minutes.
- Fluff the cooked wild rice with a fork, then stir in the sautéed mushrooms and peas.
- Add salt and pepper to taste.
- Serve hot.

Nutritional Information (Per Serving):

- *Calories: 210.*
- *Protein: 7 grams.*
- *Dietary fibre: 4g*

CHAPTER 8

Snacks And Sides That Will Keep You Satisfied.

Cucumber Sandwiches.

- _**Servings: Two.**_
- _**Prep time: 10 minutes.**_

Ingredients:

- Four pieces of whole grain bread.
- One cucumber, thinly sliced
- 2 tablespoons cream cheese (low-fat).
- Dill or chives as garnish (optional)

Instructions:

- Spread the cream cheese equally on the slices of bread.
- Spread the cucumber slices over two slices of bread.
- Optional garnishes include dill or chives.
- Top with the remaining bread slices, then cut each sandwich in half or quarters.
- Serve immediately, or refrigerate before serving.

Nutritional Information (Per Serving):

- *Calories:180*
- *Protein: 6 grams*
- *Dietary fibre: 3 grams*

Carrot Sticks and Hummus

- ***Servings: Two.***
- ***Prep time: 5 minutes.***

Ingredients:

- 2 large carrots peeled and sliced into sticks.
- 1/2 cup hummus.

Instructions:

- Arrange carrot sticks on a platter.
- Serve alongside a cup of hummus for dipping.
- Enjoy as a crunchy, healthful snack.

Nutritional Information (Per Serving):

- Calories: 140.
- Protein: 4 grams
- Dietary fibre: 4g

Baked Apple Chips

- *Serves: 4*
- *Prep Time: 2 hours and 15 minutes.*

Ingredients:

- Two apples, cored and thinly sliced
- One teaspoon of ground cinnamon.

Instructions:

- Pre-heat the oven to 200°F (95°C).
- Place the apple slices in a single layer on a baking sheet coated with parchment paper.
- Sprinkle the slices with cinnamon.
- Bake for 2 hours, flipping halfway through, until the slices are dry and crisp.
- Let cool before serving.

Nutritional Information (Per Serving):

- *Calories: 50.*
- *Protein: 0 grams*
- *Dietary fibre: 3 grams*

Oatmeal Raisin Cookies

- *Serving size: 12 cookies.*
- *Prep time: 25 minutes.*

Ingredients:

- One cup rolled oats.
- 3/4 cup whole wheat flour.
- 1/2 teaspoon of baking soda.
- One-half teaspoon cinnamon
- 1/4 cup unsweetened applesauce.
- 1/4 cup of honey (optional)
- 1 egg
- 1/2 teaspoon of vanilla extract.
- One-half cup raisins

Instructions:

- Preheat the oven to 350°F/175°C.
- In a bowl, combine oats, flour, baking soda, and cinnamon.
- In another bowl, combine applesauce, honey (if using), egg, and vanilla essence.
- Mix together the wet and dry ingredients, then fold in the raisins.
- Place tablespoonfuls of dough on a baking sheet coated with parchment paper.

- Bake for 10–12 minutes, or until the edges are brown.
- Cool on the baking sheet for a few minutes before transferring to a wire rack.

Nutritional Information (Per Cookie):

- Calories: 90.
- Protein: 2 grams
- Dietary fibre: 1g

Almond Butter Rice Cakes.

- **Serves: 1**
- **Prep time: 5 minutes.**

Ingredients:

- One rice cake.
- One tablespoon almond butter.
- A dash of cinnamon (optional).

Instructions:

- Spread the almond butter evenly across the rice cake.
- Add cinnamon if desired.
- Enjoy as a quick and filling snack.

Nutritional Information (Per Serving):

- *Calories: 120.*
- *Protein: 3 grams.*
- *Dietary fibre: 1g*

Honey-Glazed Walnuts.

- ***Serves: 4***
- ***Prep time: 15 minutes.***

Ingredients:

- One cup of walnuts.
- One tablespoon of honey (optional)
- A pinch of cinnamon.

Instructions:

- Preheat the oven to 350°F/175°C.
- Combine the walnuts, honey, and cinnamon in a bowl and mix until completely coated.
- Spread the walnuts onto a baking sheet lined with parchment paper.
- Bake for 10 minutes, until aromatic and lightly toasted.
- Let cool before serving.

Nutritional Information (Per Serving):

- *Calories: 190.*
- *Protein: 4 grams*
- *Dietary fibre: 2 grams*

Baked Kale Chips

- **Servings: Two.**
- **Prep time: 20 minutes.**

Ingredients:

- 1 bunch kale, stems removed, leaves torn into bite-sized pieces.
- One tablespoon of olive oil.
- Salt to taste.

Instructions:

- Preheat your oven to 300°F (150°C).
- In a large mixing basin, combine the kale, olive oil, and salt.
- Place the kale in a single layer on a baking sheet coated with parchment paper.
- Bake for 10-15 minutes, until the sides are lightly browned but not burned.

- Allow to cool completely before serving to ensure maximum crispness.

Nutritional Information (Per Serving):

- *Calories: 60.*
- *Protein: 2 grams*
- *Dietary fibre: 1g*

Greek Yogurt with Honey and Almonds.

- **Serves: 1**
- **Prep time: 5 minutes.**

Ingredients:

- 1 cup plain Greek yogurt (low-fat)
- One tablespoon of honey (optional)
- 2 tablespoons slivered almonds.

Instructions:

- Add the Greek yogurt to a bowl.
- Drizzle with honey if desired.
- Add slivered almonds on top.
- Serve immediately and relish this creamy and crispy delicacy.

Nutritional Information (Per Serving):

- *Calories:180*
- *Protein: 20 grams*
- *Dietary fibre: 2 grams*

Roasted Chickpeas.

- **Serves: 4**
- **Prep time: 40 minutes.**

Ingredients:

- 1 can (15 ounces) of chickpeas, drained, rinsed, and dried
- One tablespoon of olive oil.
- 1/2 teaspoons smoked paprika.
- Salt to taste.

Instructions:

- Preheat your oven to 400°F (200°C).
- Combine the chickpeas, olive oil, smoked paprika, and salt.
- Arrange the chickpeas on a baking sheet in a single layer.
- Roast for 30–35 minutes, stirring the pan occasionally, until crisp and brown.
- Let cool before serving.

Nutritional Information (Per Serving):

- *Calories: 120.*
- *Protein: 6 grams*
- *Dietary fibre: 5g*

Pear Slices and Cheese

- **Serves: 1**
- **Prep time: 5 minutes.**

Ingredients:

- One ripe pear, cored and sliced
- 1 ounce of sliced cheese (such as cheddar or mozzarella).

Instructions:

- Place the pear slices on a platter.
- Place one slice of cheese on top of each pear slice.
- This sweet and salty combo makes a refreshing snack.

Nutritional Information (Per Serving):

- *Calories: 150.*
- *Protein: 7 grams.*
- *Dietary fibre: 3 grams*

Pumpkin Seeds

- *Serves: 4*
- *Preparation time: 1 hour 10 minutes.*

Ingredients:

- One cup raw pumpkin seed.
- One teaspoon of olive oil.
- One pinch of salt.

Instructions:

- Preheat your oven to 300°F (150°C).
- Combine the pumpkin seeds, olive oil, and salt.
- Arrange the seeds on a baking sheet in a single layer.
- Bake for approximately 45 minutes, stirring regularly, until brown and crispy.
- Let cool before serving.

Nutritional Information (Per Serving):

- *Calories:180*
- *Protein: 9 grams.*
- *Dietary fibre: 2 grams*

Rice Pudding with Cinnamon

- *Serves: 4*
- *Prep time: 45 minutes.*

Ingredients:

- 1/2 cup of uncooked white rice.
- 2 cups milk (or non-dairy alternative)
- 1/4 cup of sugar (optional)
- One-half teaspoon cinnamon
- 1/2 teaspoon of vanilla extract.

Instructions:

- In a saucepan, mix the rice and milk. Bring to a boil.
- Reduce the heat to low, cover, and cook for 30-35 minutes, stirring periodically, until the rice is cooked and the milk has been absorbed.
- Remove from the heat and mix in the sugar, cinnamon, and vanilla extract.
- Serve warm or chilled in the refrigerator before serving.

Nutritional Information (Per Serving):

- *Calories: 150.*
- *Protein: 4 grams*
- *Dietary fibre: 0 grams*

Homemade Granola Bars

- ***Servings: eight bars.***
- ***Prep time: 35 minutes.***

Ingredients:

- Two cups rolled oats.
- 1/4 cup of honey (optional)
- One-quarter cup almond butter
- 1/2 cup chopped almonds.
- 1/2 cup dried cranberries.

Instructions:

- Preheat the oven to 350°F/175°C.
- In a bowl, combine the oats, honey, almond butter, almonds, and dried cranberries.
- Firmly press the mixture into a prepared 8-inch square baking tray.
- Bake for 20-25 minutes, or until the edges turn golden brown.
- Allow to cool completely before cutting into bars.

Nutritional Information (Per Bar):

- *Calories: 200.*
- *Protein: 6 grams*
- *Dietary fibre: 3 grams*

Melon Balls

- ***Servings: Two.***
- ***Prep time: 10 minutes.***

Ingredients:

- 1/2 cantaloupe.
- 1/2 honeydew melon.

Instructions:

- Using a melon baller, scoop out balls of cantaloupe and honeydew melon.
- Combine the melon balls in a basin and refrigerate in the fridge.
- Serve chilled for a refreshing and hydrating snack.

Nutritional Information (Per Serving):

- Calories: 60.
- Protein: 1 gram.
- Dietary fibre: 1g

Whole Grain Crackers with Avocado Spread

- *Servings: Two.*
- *Prep time: 10 minutes.*

Ingredients:

- Four whole grain crackers.
- One ripe avocado.
- Add lemon juice to taste.
- Salt to taste.

Instructions:

- In a bowl, mash the avocado and add the lemon juice and salt.
- Spread the avocado mixture over whole grain crackers.
- Serve immediately and enjoy this creamy, crispy snack.

Nutritional Information (Per Serving):

- Calories: 140.
- Protein: 2 grams
- Dietary fibre: 5g

CHAPTER 9

BONUS

28-Day Meal Plan

Week 1

Day 1:

- Breakfast: Banana oatmeal smoothie.
- Lunch: Grilled chicken salad with balsamic vinaigrette.
- Dinner is baked salmon with dill and lemon.
- Snack: Cucumber sandwiches.

Day 2:

- Breakfast: Pear and Spinach Green Smoothie
- Lunch: Baked sweet potatoes with cottage cheese.
- Dinner: Grilled turkey burgers and oatmeal.
- Snack: Carrot sticks and hummus.

Day 3:

- Breakfast: Ginger-infused overnight oats.
- Lunch: turkey and spinach wrap with avocado.
- Dinner: Vegetable stir-fry with ginger sauce.
- Snack: baked apple chips.

Day 4:

- Breakfast: Avocado toast with poached egg.
- Lunch: Butternut squash soup.
- Dinner: Lemon-herb roasted chicken
- Snack: oatmeal raisin cookies.

Day 5:

- Breakfast: Quinoa porridge with apples and cinnamon.
- Lunch is Quinoa Tabbouleh Salad.
- Dinner: Baked cod with steamed broccoli.
- Snack: Almond butter rice cakes.

Day 6:

- Breakfast: Almond butter and banana pancakes
- Lunch: Rice paper rolls with mango and mint.
- Dinner: herb-crusted tilapia with asparagus.
- Snack: Honey-glazed walnuts.

Day 7:

- Breakfast: Baked pears with honey and walnuts.
- Lunch: Baked falafel with Tahini Sauce.
- Dinner: Stuffed bell peppers with quinoa.
- Snack: baked kale chips.

Week 2

Day 8:

- Breakfast: Carrot and ginger juice.

- Lunch: Lentil salad with cucumbers and herbs.

- Dinner: Chicken and vegetable skewers

- Snack: Greek yogurt with honey and almonds.

Day 9:

- Breakfast: Multigrain waffles with maple syrup.

- Lunch: Roasted beet and carrot salad.

- Dinner: Eggplant Parmesan with Low Acid Tomato Sauce.

- Snack: roasted chickpeas.

Day 10:

- Breakfast: Baked oatmeal cups with blueberries.

- Lunch: Cauliflower Rice Stir-Fry.

- Dinner: Roasted turkey breast with sweet potatoes.

- Snack: Pear slices and cheese.

Day 11:

- Breakfast: Chia Seed Pudding and Almond Milk

- Lunch: Broccoli and cheese stuffed potatoes.

- Dinner: Grilled shrimp with garlic and herbs.

- Snack: Pumpkin seeds.

Day 12:

- Breakfast: Whole wheat banana muffins.
- Lunch: Zucchini noodles with pesto.
- Dinner is Seared Scallops with Polenta.
- Snack: rice pudding with cinnamon.

Day 13:

- Breakfast: savoury oatmeal with avocado.
- Lunch: Grilled fish tacos with cabbage slaw.
- Dinner: vegetarian lasagna with spinach and ricotta.
- Snack: homemade granola bars.

Day 14:

- Breakfast: Apple Cinnamon Quinoa
- Lunch: Vegetable Quiche with Oat Crust.
- Dinner: Pork tenderloin with roasted apples.
- Snack: Melon balls.

Week 3

Day 15:

- Breakfast: Yogurt parfait with mixed berries.
- Lunch is Soba Noodle Salad with Edamame.
- Dinner is wild rice pilaf with mushrooms and peas.
- Snack: Whole grain crackers and avocado spread.

(Repeat the cycle on Days 16–21)

Week 4

Day 22:

- Breakfast: Banana oatmeal smoothie.
- Lunch: Grilled chicken salad with balsamic vinaigrette.
- Dinner is baked salmon with dill and lemon.
- Snack: Cucumber sandwiches.

Day 23:

- Breakfast: Pear and Spinach Green Smoothie
- Lunch: Baked sweet potatoes with cottage cheese.
- Dinner: Grilled turkey burgers and oatmeal.
- Snack: carrot sticks and hummus.

Day 24:

- Breakfast: Ginger-infused overnight oats.
- Lunch: turkey and spinach wrap with avocado.
- Dinner: Vegetable stir-fry with ginger sauce.
- Snack: baked apple chips.

Day 25:

- Breakfast: Avocado toast with poached egg.
- Lunch: Butternut squash soup.
- Dinner: Lemon-herb roasted chicken
- Snack: oatmeal raisin cookies.

Day 26:

- Breakfast: Quinoa porridge with apples and cinnamon.
- Lunch is Quinoa Tabbouleh Salad.
- Dinner: Baked cod with steamed broccoli.
- Snack: Almond butter rice cakes.

Day 27:

- Breakfast: Almond butter and banana pancakes
- Lunch: Rice paper rolls with mango and mint.
- Dinner: herb-crusted tilapia with asparagus.
- Snack: Honey-glazed walnuts.

Day 28:

- Breakfast: Baked pears with honey and walnuts.
- Lunch: Baked falafel with Tahini Sauce.
- Dinner: Stuffed bell peppers with quinoa.
- Snack: baked kale chips.

Each day is designed to deliver balanced nutrients while maintaining an acid reflux-friendly diet. Remember to modify the recipes and portion quantities to meet your individual nutritional needs and tastes, and speak with a healthcare provider if you have any special dietary concerns. Enjoy your meals!

Shopping List

Fruit and Vegetable

- Apples.
- Bananas
- Blueberries.
- Cantaloupe
- Carrots.
- Cauliflower
- Cucumber.
- Honeydew melon.
- Kale
- Lemons.
- Mangos.
- Mixed Berries
- Pears.
- Red onions.
- Spinach.
- Sweet Potatoes
- Zucchini

Proteins

- Chicken breasts.
- Cod fillets.
- Eggs
- Ground turkey.
- Salmon fillets
- Shrimp.
- Tilapia fillets.
- Turkey breast.

Dairy and Non-dairy Alternatives

- Almond Milk
- Cheddar cheese (low fat)
- Cottage Cheese.
- Greek yogurt (plain, low fat)
- mozzarella cheese (low-fat)
- Parmesan cheese.
- Ricotta cheese (low fat)

Grains and legumes

- Black beans.
- Brown Rice
- Chickpeas.
- Corn tortillas.

- Edamame.
- Lentils.
- Oats
- Quinoa
- Rice cakes
- Rolled Oats
- Soba noodles.
- Wholegrain bread.
- Whole Grain Crackers
- Whole wheat flour.

Nuts, seeds, and dried fruit

- Almonds.
- Almond Butter
- Chia Seeds
- Dried Cranberries.
- Honey (Optional)
- Pumpkin Seeds
- Raisins
- Walnuts.

Herbs, spices, and condiments.

- Balsamic vinegar.
- Basil.
- Cinnamon.

- Dill
- Garlic.
- Ginger.
- Maple syrup.
- Olive Oil.
- Oregano.
- Parsley.
- Sesame oil.
- Soy sauce (low sodium).
- Tahini.
- Thyme.
- Vanilla Extract

Miscellaneous

- Baked soda
- Cornstarch.
- Honey (Optional)
- Low-acid tomato sauce.
- Parchment Paper
- Rice Paper
- Sugar (Optional)

Remember to alter the numbers based on the number of servings you intend to make, and to check for any personal dietary restrictions or preferences. Happy cooking

CONCLUSION

As we come to the end of this guide to an acid reflux-friendly diet, I hope you found the journey through each recipe and meal plan to be not only informative but also beneficial to your health and well-being.

Each person's road to managing acid reflux is unique, and regular adherence to the dietary recommendations indicated in this book can be a cornerstone in creating a life with fewer symptoms and more enjoyment of the foods you love.

Consistency is essential in any dietary adjustment, and I sincerely hope that the dishes and advice presented here become a regular part of your daily routine. Remember that small, sustainable adjustments can lead to long-term health advantages.

I advise you to view this acid reflux-friendly diet as a positive lifestyle adjustment that provides a diversity of Flavors while keeping your comfort in mind.

While this book is useful as a guide, it is important to remember that specific advice from healthcare professionals is priceless. Your experience with acid reflux is unique, and a healthcare expert may provide specialized recommendations based on your specific health profile, ensuring that the diet you follow is as effective and beneficial as possible.

If this book has served you well, added new tastes to your table, and improved your health, I would appreciate it if you could share your experience. Your feedback is not only a beacon for others facing the hardships of acid reflux, but it is also a vital reflection that can help shape future versions of the book.

Thank you for making this book a part of your culinary journey.

May your meals be delicious, your health be vibrant, and your days be full with the pleasures of good food and well-being.